BOOST YOUR IMMUNITY

The Ultimate Guide to stay healthy and live longer

ALICE BEN

TABLE OF CONTENTS

- **Introduction**
1. **Maintain Personal Hygiene**
2. **Quit Smoking**
3. **Keep Hydrated**
4. **Minimize Stress**
5. **Set Up Sleep Routine**
6. **Take Vitamins**
7. **Working Out Regularly**
8. **Practice Deep Breathing Techniques**
9. **Employ Positive Thinking/Attitude**
10. **Healthy Eating**
11. **Maintain Healthy Weight**

INTRODUCTION

When it comes to protecting our health, our immune system plays a vital role. We all want to take steps to ensure our immunity is as strong as possible, and there are many different strategies we can use to boost our immunity. From dietary changes to lifestyle adjustments, there are a multitude of ways to give our immune system the support it needs to function at its best. To help make sense of it all, a great resource is a book that outlines different ways to boost your immunity. This guide will provide an overview of the most effective strategies to ensure your immune system is working optimally.

CHAPTER 1

MAINTAIN PERSONAL HYGIENE

Both physical and mental health can benefit from good personal cleanliness.
Maintaining a clean, healthy external body requires good personal hygiene. Maintaining both physical and mental wellness depends on it. People with poor personal hygiene give the body the perfect conditions for germs to flourish, making them more susceptible to sickness. A person with poor personal hygiene may experience social isolation and loneliness as a result of people avoiding them.

Maintaining appropriate cleanliness is crucial for our general health since without it, we would become ill and be unable to carry out our regular tasks. Without following excellent cleanliness practices, no one can be in good health. We come into contact with a variety of viruses, germs, bacteria, and other pollutants every day that can harm our health, but if we practice good hygiene, we can avoid being sick. You must learn how to incorporate good personal hygiene practices into your daily routine if you want to progress as a person and keep your standing in society. Here are some pointers for maintaining complete personal hygiene.

PERSONAL HYGIENE TYPES

1. Dental care
Practicing good dental hygiene goes beyond maintaining pearly whites. Gum disease and cavities can both be avoided with regular oral hygiene practice. Additionally, it can stop the foul breath.

2. Body hygiene
The average person's body has several million sweat glands. A scent or body odor is produced when bacteria decompose sweat. Washing the body will get rid of the bacteria that make you smell bad and avoid skin irritation. Hair washing eliminates grease and keeps one looking clean and young.

3. Washing hands

One of the best ways to stop the transmission of communicable diseases is by regular hand washing. The Centers for Disease Control and Prevention (CDC)Trusted Source advises washing hands at specific times such as; before, during, and after handling anyone who is vomiting or having diarrhea, before and after treating a cut or wound, before and after going to the bathroom, after changing diapers or cleaning up a child who has used the toilet, after blowing one's nose, coughing, or sneezing, and after touching trash or unclean surfaces.

4. Nails Hygiene

The transmission of bacteria may be aided by the dirt and germs that fingernails may store. Keeping your nails short can help lower your risk of contracting an infection since dirt and germs can accumulate more easily under longer nails. One of the greatest ways to make sure that no dirt can gather underneath the nails is to trim them with sanitized equipment and keep them short. A person's hand cleaning routine may include using a nail brush to scrub the area under their nails.

5. Genital hygiene
Tampons, pads, and other sanitary items should be changed regularly. It's also necessary to wash your hands before and after. Because vaginas are self-cleaning, using soap to clean them can upset their normal bacterial balance and result in infections. Only once per day does the vulva (the exterior of the vagina) need to be cleaned with light soap and water. Uncircumcised men can clean their penis by gently pulling back the foreskin and bathing the area beneath with warm water or soap.

TIPS FOR HYGIENE ROUTINE

1. Setting reminders
Set a reminder on your phone if you struggle to remember to take a shower, wash your hair, trim your nails, or brush your teeth. You'll be prompted to complete the task by the cue, and eventually, you'll start doing it on your own.

2. Use signs
A reminder to wash your hands after using the restroom should be hung in the bathroom. Make a small sign to remind you to wash your hands before eating by the plates or bowls in the kitchen. These cues can help you remember things and develop better routines. They can assist your kids as well as you.

3. Getting better with practice
A new habit takes time to develop. Make a new habit your top priority and start it at the beginning of the week. For a week or two, put it to use. Add a new one once you're comfortable with the current one. You'll develop the habits you want to have over time.

CONCLUSION
A lifetime of learning and practice is required to develop good personal hygiene practices. These self-care practices are beneficial for both your physical and mental well-being.

CHAPTER 2

QUIT SMOKING

People who smoke frequently begin because their friends or family do. However, people continue to smoke because nicotine, one of the compounds in cigarettes and smokeless tobacco, becomes addictive.

Nicotine has stimulant and depressive properties. That indicates that it first raises heart rate and causes people to feel more alert. The result is melancholy and exhaustion. People yearn for another cigarette to boost them back up again because of their despair and exhaustion as well as the chemical withdrawal from nicotine. According to some experts, tobacco's nicotine is just as addictive as heroin or cocaine.

Unfortunately, as the 6.9 million smokers in the UK will attest, it can be challenging to quit this specific habit! No matter how hard you try, nicotine's addictiveness continues luring you back for more.

Breaking the cycle of addiction and effectively reprogramming the brain to cease craving nicotine are two key components of quitting smoking. Smokers who wish to stop need to have a strategy in place to combat cravings and triggers to be successful.

The advantages of stopping smoking might start as soon as an hour following the final cigarette. The sooner a smoker gives up, the faster their risk of developing cancer, heart disease, lung disease, and other smoking-related illnesses is reduced.

The advantages are almost immediate. A smoker's body starts to recuperate as soon as they stop smoking in the following ways:

AT ONE HOUR.

The heart rate decreases and returns to normal in as little as 20 minutes after the final cigarette is smoked. Circulation may start to improve as blood pressure starts to decline.

12 HOURS LATER

Carbon monoxide, a chemical included in cigarette smoke, is one of many known poisons found in cigarettes. High concentrations of this gas, which blocks oxygen from reaching the lungs and blood, can be dangerous or even fatal. Suffocation from a lack of oxygen can happen when inhaled in high dosages over a short time.

The body rids itself of the extra carbon monoxide from cigarettes in just 12 hours without smoking. The body's oxygen levels rise when the level of carbon monoxide returns to normal.

AFTER A DAY

After just one day of quitting smoking, the risk of having a heart attack starts to go down. Smoking increases the risk of coronary heart disease by lowering good cholesterol, which makes it more difficult to engage in heart-healthy exercise. Smoking also increases blood clotting and blood pressure, which boosts the risk of stroke.

A person's blood pressure starts to decline as soon as 1 day after quitting smoking, lowering the risk of heart disease from smoking-induced high blood pressure. A person's oxygen levels will have increased during this brief period, making exercise and physical activity easier to perform and encouraging heart-healthy habits.

IN TWO DAYS

The nerve endings responsible for taste and smell are harmed by smoking. A person may experience a more acute sense of smell and more vivid tastes in as little as 2 days after quitting as these nerves heal.

IN THIRD DAYS

The nicotine levels in a person's body are depleted 3 days after they stop smoking. Although having no nicotine in the body is healthier, the early depletion of nicotine might result in withdrawal symptoms. Most people endure moodiness and irritability, excruciating headaches, and cravings three days after stopping as their bodies adjust.

AFTER A MONTH

One can see improvement in lung function in as little as one month. Former smokers may experience a decrease in coughing and shortness of breath as their lungs recover and their lung capacity increases. Former smokers may experience an improvement in their physical stamina and a fresh capacity for cardiovascular exercises like running and jumping.

3 TO 6 MONTHS LATER

Circulation gets better for several months after you stop smoking.

NINE MONTHS LATER

The lungs have considerably repaired themselves nine months after stopping. The lungs' fragile cilia, which resemble tiny hairs, have healed from the damage caused by cigarette smoke. These features aid in removing mucus from the lungs and ward against infections. Because the healed cilia can perform their function more readily at this time, many ex-smokers experience a decrease in the frequency of lung infections.

ONE YEAR LATER

A person's risk of developing coronary heart disease is cut in half one year after stopping smoking. After one year, this risk will continue to decrease.

IN FIVE YEARS

Numerous well-known toxins found in cigarettes restrict the arteries and blood vessels. The risk of blood clots is likewise raised by these same poisons.

The body has sufficiently healed itself after quitting smoking for five years for the arteries and blood vessels to start to enlarge once more. The blood is less prone to clot as a result of this expansion, which reduces the risk of stroke.

Over the following ten years, as the body gets more and better at healing, the chance of stroke will continue to decline.

IN TEN YEARS

Compared to someone who continues to smoke, a person's odds of developing lung cancer and dying from it are nearly cut in half after ten years. Pancreatic, oral, and throat cancer risks have been dramatically decreased.

15 YEARS LATER

The risk of getting coronary heart disease is comparable to that of a non-smoker 15 years after quitting smoking. The chance of acquiring pancreatic cancer has also decreased to match that of a non-smoker.

UPON 20 YEARS

The chance of dying from smoking-related conditions, such as cancer and lung disease, decreases to that of someone who has never smoked in their life after 20 years. Additionally, the chance of developing pancreatic cancer has decreased to that of a non-smoker.

SMOKE QUITTING TIPS

1. Skip the danger areas:
When you first quit, your mind will search for any justification to light up again. Therefore, it's critical to recognize and stay away from places and times where you're accustomed to smoking (like the bar or while drinking your morning coffee).

You can prevent potential triggers from leading to relapse by consciously avoiding these circumstances and/or having a strategy in place to act differently. Play games with friends at home, use a pen to keep your fingers busy, etc.

2. Get distracted:
The desires that are certain to arise can be resisted in the short term by using distractions. You can distract yourself from the need to smoke by finding something else to concentrate on. It is easy to use but efficient.

You decide how to divert your attention, although exercise is one strategy that is frequently suggested.

Running up the stairs, doing pushups, or going for a stroll can all be great ways to divert your attention while also improving your physical health. If that doesn't work, try journaling, doing housework, or playing with the dog—anything to get your mind off of smoking!

3. Test your self-hypnosis skills:
Another tried-and-true method for quitting smoking swiftly is self-hypnosis. You become more driven, open to change, and empowered when you self-induce hypnosis. As a result, quitting the habit becomes simpler. Not like what you see in the movies, hypnosis doesn't work like that. It's not magic. Simply said, you're in a very relaxed state, which is typically attained by visualization and breathing techniques.

You listen to and/or repeat to yourself pertinent statements and affirmations on quitting smoking when you're in this calm, focused state. Your subconscious mind gets rewired as a result of the audio hypnosis, and you soon start thinking, feeling, and behaving like a non-smoker.

CONCLUSION

Smoking is a bad habit that can cause serious health issues and even death. After quitting smoking, a person's body will gradually begin to naturally mend and regain the vitality of a non-smoker. Some effects, including reduced blood pressure, are seen right away. It takes time for other effects, such as the likelihood of getting lung cancer, heart disease, or another lung condition, to diminish to those of a non-smoker.

However, every year of cessation reduces risks and enhances general health, making giving up smoking a wise decision for anyone who developed the habit.

CHAPTER 3

KEEP HYDRATED

Water is vital to life and is necessary for survival. Most of what makes up your body is water. It makes up just over half of a woman's body and almost two-thirds of a man's. Your body needs water to do several things, like flush out waste materials in your urine, lubricate your joints, carry nutrients throughout your body, and regulate your body temperature. Your skin may even look better as a result of it. Drinking water provides a variety of advantages, such as:

1. Controlling body temperature internally
2. Food metabolization and control of hunger
3. Joint lubrication
4. Flushing body waste
5. Generating enough saliva

Dehydration can cause reduced renal function, imbalanced electrolytes, and other problems if you don't drink enough water. Delaying taking a drink until you're thirsty is crucial because of this. Instead, take control of your hydration and establish enduring habits to maintain energy levels throughout the day. We get around 20% of the fluid we need each day from our food and the remainder from the liquids we drink.

Depending on the sex you were given at birth, you need to drink a certain amount of water. The U.S. National Academies of Science, Engineering, and Medicine recommends that males consume 3.7 liters (or 16 cups) of fluid per day and women consume 2.7 liters (or 11 cups). If you work out, perspire, or are ill, you should consume even more water (diarrhea, vomiting, fever).

It is possible to consume too much water, although it is uncommon. A water surplus can be fatal, particularly for people with heart disease or electrolyte imbalances. The best course of action is to discuss with your doctor how much water is optimal for you to consume given your activity level and body type.

HOW TO REMAIN HYDRATED

1. Sip a minimum of 1 glass of water before each meal. An excellent technique to stay hydrated is to drink water while eating. Water consumption before, during, or after a meal not only makes it convenient but also promotes digestion. Water and other hydrating liquids can be consumed to aid with food digestion and nutrient absorption. Additionally, water acts as a stool softener, assisting in the reduction of constipation. Make sure to drink a glass of water along with your meal, even if you choose to indulge in tea, juice, or soda.

2. Establish clear objectives and monitor your fluid intake.
You could be asking yourself, "What's the magic number?" or "How much water should I drink each day?" No single formula works for everyone, is the

response. It will be easier for you to determine how much water to consume each day if you are more aware of your body's need for fluids.

3. Make it Tasty!
Unfortunately, water has poor taste compared to other beverages like coffee, tea, soda, and juice, which are far more enticing. Today's grocery store shelves are crowded with countless options, which leads many consumers to select beverages that are high in sugar, artificial sweeteners, and empty calories. But here are some suggestions for spicing up your fluid intake while keeping it tasty, attractive, and thirst-quenching.
i. Slices of orange, lime, or lemon added to water
These citrus fruits will give your water a revitalizing flavor and enhance the aesthetics of your glass. They also include a significant amount of vitamin C, a key antioxidant and immunity booster. To us, this situation is a win-win! These can enhance the flavor of your water and make it even more refreshing by adding a natural, distinct flavor. It will also appear lovely!

ii. Fruit pieces frozen in ice cube trays
Consider freezing blackberries or raspberries in water-filled ice cube trays. After that, put the fruit-filled ice in a cup, add water, and drink up! We refer to it as creatively hydrating, however, some may call it art.
iii. Consider sparkling water
If you like bubbles, sip on seltzer or sparkling water. While still being calorie-free, it quenches the thirst and offers a refreshing contrast from flat water. Although you don't feel as though you're drinking water, it nevertheless has hydrating properties.

4. Always have a reusable water bottle with you everywhere you go.
Reduce, reuse, and recycle are what we live by! Reusable water bottles are not only an excellent method to stay hydrated throughout the day but also a terrific fashion statement (not to mention they are great for the environment and limit plastic waste).

5. Sip water as soon as you wake up.

What do you do first thing in the morning? Obviously after pressing the snooze button. using your phone to check social media? Go to the restroom to clean your teeth? Think about drinking a glass of water to start your day. A glass of water in the morning helps to balance your lymphatic system by flushing your stomach. Your immune system will be supported, helping to keep you from becoming sick as frequently. Drinking water first thing in the morning helps your body wake up and stimulates your digestive system.

After a night of sleep, drinking water helps you rehydrate and gets your day started on the right foot. Start your day hydrated if you want to stay hydrated.

6. Consume fruits and vegetables with a high water content, like melons, berries, lettuce, and celery. Although drinking water is necessary, you can also keep hydrated by eating foods high in water. To be hydrated, many people don't necessarily need to consume a lot of water. You won't have difficulty remaining hydrated as long as you're consuming

enough water-rich foods (including lettuce, celery, cucumbers, berries, and melons) and drinking water when you're thirsty. Peaches, skim milk, cottage cheese, as well as broths and soups, are additional WATER-RICH FOODS.

7. Examine the color of your urine.
Some people monitor their urine's color throughout the day to make sure it is clear or pale. Some people's dark yellow urine could be a sign of dehydration.

CONCLUSION

Despite the inconvenience of constantly drinking water, the numerous advantages for your physical and mental health make it worthwhile. That's why we provided you with simple, long-lasting advice on how to stay hydrated throughout your daily activities. With these pointers, we hope to inspire you to develop hydration routines that will improve both your physical and emotional health.

CHAPTER 4

MINIMIZE STRESS

Many people frequently endure stress and worry. Millions of American people claim to experience everyday stress or worry. Many people experience stress daily. Everyday stresses such as those related to work, family, health, and finances can often lead to higher stress levels.

Additionally, a person's susceptibility to stress is influenced by factors including heredity, the amount of social support they receive, their coping mechanisms, and their personality, thus some people are more likely to experience stress than others.

Illnesses are significantly influenced by stress. One in three people reports feeling extremely stressed out in their daily lives, which raises the possibility of hazardous viruses already present in our bodies becoming active. Stress impairs our body's capacity to produce antibodies that can fight off foreign substances. Stressful events and everyday stress can be harmful to our immune systems. Your immune system will develop stronger and you will live longer if you can fit more stress-reduction activities into your life.

WAYS TO REDUCE STRESS

1. Increase your level of exercise
Consistently moving your body can help if you're feeling stressed. In a 6-week study involving 185 university students, aerobic exercise on two days a week significantly decreased both overall reported stress and perceived stress resulting from uncertainty. Additionally, the exercise program greatly enhanced self-reported depression

Numerous other researchers have demonstrated that physical activity improves mood and lowers stress levels, whereas sedentary behavior may increase stress, negatively impact mood, and interfere with sleep. Additionally, regular exercise has been shown to lessen the symptoms of common mental health issues including depression and anxiety. Start slowly if you aren't already active, perhaps with some riding or walking. Selecting an enjoyable hobby can improve your likelihood of sustaining it over time.

2. Maintain a balanced diet

Every area of your health, including your mental health, is impacted by your nutrition. According to studies, persons who consume a diet heavy in ultra-processed foods and added sugar are more likely to perceive their stress levels as being higher. Chronic stress may cause you to overeat and gravitate toward very tasty meals, which could be detrimental to your general health and mood.

Moreso, eating too few nutrient-dense whole foods may increase your risk of falling short on nutrients like magnesium and B vitamins, which are crucial for controlling stress and mood. Your body can be better nourished if you consume fewer highly processed meals and beverages and more whole foods like vegetables, fruits, legumes, seafood, nuts, and seeds.

Thus, you might become more stress-resistant as a result.

3. Reduce screen and phone time.
For many people, smartphones, computers, and tablets are essential components of daily life. Even while these gadgets are frequently necessary, overusing them can lead to stress.

Numerous studies have connected elevated levels of stress and mental health concerns with excessive smartphone use and "iPhone addiction." In general, excessive screen usage is linked to lower psychological well-being and higher levels of stress in both adults and children. Additionally, screen usage may harm sleep, which could result in greater stress.

4. Consider Supplements
The stress response and mood management of your body are significantly influenced by several vitamins and minerals. As a result, a vitamin shortage may have an impact on your mental health and capacity to handle stress.

Furthermore, some research indicates that specific nutritional supplements may aid in lowering stress and enhancing mood. For instance, your magnesium levels may drop if you experience persistent stress. It's crucial to make sure you get enough of this mineral every day because it's crucial for your body's reaction to stress. Magnesium supplementation has been demonstrated to reduce chronic stress in adults.

300 mg of this mineral per day was found to significantly lower stress levels in an 8-week study of 264 individuals with low magnesium levels. This dosage of magnesium worked considerably better when combined with vitamin B6. It has also been demonstrated that other supplements, such as Rhodiola, ashwagandha, B vitamins, and L-theanine, can also aid in stress reduction. However, not everyone may benefit from or feel safe using dietary supplements. If you're interested in using supplements to lessen stress, speak with a healthcare provider.

5. Limit your caffeine consumption

Your central nervous system is stimulated by caffeine, a substance present in coffee, tea, chocolate, and energy drinks. Anxiety symptoms may worsen and grow stronger if you consume too much.

Furthermore, excessive use may interfere with your ability to sleep. As a result, tension and anxiety symptoms could worsen. The maximum amount of caffeine that each person can tolerate varies. Consider reducing your intake of caffeine by substituting decaffeinated herbal tea or water for coffee or energy drinks if you find that it makes you jittery or anxious.

Although numerous studies demonstrate the health benefits of coffee when consumed in moderation, it is advised to limit daily caffeine intake to 400 mg, or around 4-5 cups (0.9–1.2 L) of coffee. It's crucial to take into account your tolerance because those who are sensitive to caffeine may suffer heightened anxiety and tension even after eating considerably less caffeine than this.

6. Spend time with loved ones.
You might benefit from the social support of friends
and family to get through difficult times and deal
with stress. In a study of 163 Latinx college students,
loneliness, depressive symptoms, and perceived
stress were all connected with lower levels of support
from friends, family, and romantic partners.

Your total mental health depends on the strength of
your social support network. Social support groups
could be useful if you're feeling lonely and don't have
friends or family to rely on. Think about joining a
club, a sports team, or volunteering for an
organization that matters to you.

7. Set limits and develop the ability to refuse.
Some pressures are out of your control, but not all of
them. Overcommitting yourself could result in a
higher stress level and less time available for
self-care. Being in charge of your personal life can
help you feel less stressed and safeguard your mental
health.

Saying "no" more frequently might be one method to do this. This is particularly important to remember if you frequently take on more than you can manage because juggling multiple obligations might make you feel overburdened. Stress levels can be decreased by being cautious about what you take on and saying "no" to things that would unnecessarily add to your workload.

Setting boundaries is a smart method to safeguard your well-being, particularly with those that increase your stress levels. Simply asking a friend or family member not to drop by unexpectedly or canceling standing plans with a friend who tends to stir up trouble will accomplish this.

8. Develop the habit of staying on task.
Keeping track of your priorities and avoiding procrastination are two other ways to manage your stress. Your productivity could suffer if you procrastinate, leaving you with little time to make up for the lost time. Stress might result from this, which is bad for your health and the quality of your sleep.

Procrastination and elevated stress levels were connected in a Chinese study of 140 medical students. The study also linked more unfavorable parenting practices, such as discipline and rejection, with procrastination and delayed stress reactions.

Developing the practice of creating a to-do list that is prioritized may be helpful if you frequently procrastinate. Set reasonable deadlines for yourself and proceed through the list. Give yourself undisturbed time to work on the tasks that must be completed today. Multitasking or switching between things can be stressful in and of itself.

9. Attend a yoga session

Yoga has gained popularity as a form of exercise and stress reduction for people of all ages. While there are many different types of yoga, they all aim to bring the body and the mind together by raising body and breath awareness.

Yoga has been shown in numerous studies to aid with stress management and the signs of anxiety and depression. Additionally, it can support psychological health. These advantages appear to be connected to how your neurological system and stress response are affected.

Yoga has been shown to increase levels of gamma-aminobutyric acid, a neurotransmitter that is low in those who suffer from mood disorders, while decreasing cortisol, blood pressure, and heart rate.

10. Incorporate mindfulness.
The term "mindfulness" refers to techniques that keep you focused on the present. Both mindfulness meditation and mindfulness-based cognitive therapy (MBCT), a subset of cognitive behavioral therapy, are methods for reducing the stress that make use of mindfulness.

Consistently meditating, even for little durations, may improve your mood and lessen the signs of stress and worry. Numerous books, apps, and websites can teach you the fundamentals of meditation if you want to give it a try.

11. Spend time in nature

More time spent outside could help lower stress. Studies have shown that being in nature and spending time in green areas like parks and forests are excellent strategies to manage stress.

According to a meta-analysis of 14 studies, college-aged individuals may benefit psychologically and physically by spending as little as 10 minutes in a natural environment. These markers include perceived stress and happiness. Although hiking and camping are excellent possibilities, some people don't like them or don't have access to them. You can look for green areas like neighborhood parks, arboretums, and botanical gardens even if you reside in a city.

12. Practice inhaling deeply

Your sympathetic nervous system is activated by mental stress, putting your body into a fight-or-flight response. Stress hormones cause physical symptoms like a faster heartbeat, shallower breathing, and constricted blood vessels during this reaction.The parasympathetic nerve system, which regulates the relaxation response, may be activated with the aid of deep breathing exercises. Diaphragmatic breathing, abdominal breathing, belly breathing, and timed respiration are all examples of deep breathing exercises.

The purpose of deep breathing is to slow down and deepen your breathing by concentrating your mind on it. Your tummy rises and your lungs fully expand when you take a deep breath through your nose. This lowers your heart rate and makes you feel calmer.

13. Bond with your pet.
Having a pet may help you feel happier and less stressed. Your body releases oxytocin when you pat or snuggle a pet, a hormone associated with happiness.

Also, research indicates that pet owners, particularly those who own dogs, tend to have higher levels of life satisfaction, better self-esteem, lower levels of loneliness and anxiety, and happier dispositions. A pet can give you a purpose, keep you busy, and provide companionship, all of which can reduce stress.

CONCLUSION

Although stress is an inevitable aspect of life, it can have negative effects on your physical and emotional well-being if it persists. Fortunately, there are many scientifically supported techniques that can help you lower stress and enhance your overall psychological health.

Effective strategies include exercise, mindfulness, spending time with a pet, reducing screen time, and spending more time outside.

CHAPTER 5

SET UP A SLEEP ROUTINE

It is essential to get enough sleep to ensure that your immune system is operating at its peak. Experts recommend getting between 7-8 hours of sleep each night is essential as our immune system needs to function properly. During this time, the body repairs itself, and getting enough sleep helps to improve the effectiveness of your white blood cell defenses against diseases. Furthermore, getting enough sleep can also reduce common cold and flu-related symptoms.

Therefore, it is important to try and establish a nighttime routine that allows you to have a restful night's sleep and receive your recommended number of hours. This will ensure that your overall health and well-being are supported. Additionally, by making sure you get 8 hours of sleep each night, you will ensure that your immune system remains efficient and effective in fighting off any potential illnesses or diseases.

Regardless of what else is going on in the world, nighttime habits frequently affect the quality of sleep. Your ability to go to sleep and stay asleep each night might be significantly impacted by your evening activities. Numerous negative health effects of insufficient sleep are possible, many of which you would worry about while lying awake. To discover potential issue areas and establish a new pattern that encourages better sleep, try looking into your pre-bedtime routines if you regularly struggle to obtain enough restful sleep.

Sure, you'll doze off eventually if you don't have a nighttime routine. However, no one can predict how long it will take or how soundly you will truly sleep once the lights are down. According to Rebecca Scott, research assistant professor of neurology at the NYU Langone Comprehensive Epilepsy Center—Sleep Center, "Most of us cannot fall asleep on command, but routine helps the brain realize that it's preparing for sleep." "Like other neurophysiological systems, our sleep system enjoys predictability and stability."

Why? Because stability and predictability are boring. It's serene. Dr. Rafael Pelayo, clinical professor of psychiatry and behavioral sciences at the Stanford Center for Sleep Sciences and Medicine, asserts that "routine indicates safety." We read the same story to children every night because of this.

You can get the required amount of sleep each night by creating a sleep schedule that suits you. Sleep routines are things you do every night before bed. Sleep duration and quality can both be enhanced by routines. To sustain a long-term healthy diet and exercise habits, getting a good night's sleep is crucial. The cheapest and probably most cost-effective step you can take toward well-being is getting enough sleep. You can improve your chances of getting better sleep by including even a small step before bed.

TIPS TO DEVELOP YOUR ROUTINE

1. Enjoy a Hot Bath.
Your body experiences some hormonal changes during the day as part of your sleep-wake cycle. Melatonin production is one of them, and it starts in the evening to get you ready for bed. Your core body temperature decreases concurrently.

Researchers have discovered that taking a warm bath can have a similar sedative effect to the body's natural evening dip in temperature. A warm bath might be a good idea an hour or so before bed. Your body will heat up from the water and quickly cool down as the water evaporates, making you feel exhausted and at ease.

2. Keep a journal or a to-do list.
Many people find journaling to be therapeutic and doing it in the evening before bed allows them to organize their thoughts and feelings.

If the thought of journaling intimidates you, think about beginning with a straightforward to-do list. According to one study, making a fast list of things that need to get done the next few days in the five minutes before bed considerably speeds up the onset of sleep.

3. Enjoy a little snack or tea before bed.
Before bed, eating large meals and drinking alcohol can cause indigestion, acid reflux, and wakefulness due to bathroom trips in the middle of the night. Going to bed hungry, however, can also cause stomach trouble and make it difficult to fall asleep.

By soothing your stomach with a light snack like a piece of fruit or yogurt, you can find a healthy middle ground. Cherries, grapes, strawberries, almonds, oats, and strawberries all contain a lot of melatonin. Another wonderful method for calming the mind and promoting sleep is non-caffeinated herbal teas, particularly those that contain chamomile or lavender. Just remember to use the bathroom before going to bed!

4. Establish a Regular Bedtime.

A few hours before bedtime, your brain begins to prepare for sleep as part of your natural sleep-wake cycle. You can improve that procedure by using your bedtime routine. Set a time for going to bed and waking up, then adhere to it every day. Consistently following a sleep schedule teaches your brain to become naturally sleepy at bedtime.

5. Take in some music.
62 percent of adults report using music to fall asleep. It doesn't matter what genre it is as long as you can unwind to it. Put your eyes closed and let the music soothe you and help you forget your concerns.

Ambient sounds, white noise, and pink noise are other audio genres that can help fall asleep. White noise may make you fall asleep more quickly by masking other sounds, whereas pink noise, such as rain or waves, has been demonstrated to increase the quality of sleep. On Spotify and smart home gadgets like Alexa, you may find tracks for various kinds of white noise.

6. Don't Touch the Electronics.
Contrary to popular belief, relaxing with your favorite
Netflix show or scrolling through Instagram does not
work. Strong blue light is emitted by all electronic
gadgets, including computers, televisions, cell
phones, and tablets. By flooding your brain with blue
light while using these devices, you can deceive it into
believing that it is daytime. Your brain attempts to
stay awake by suppressing the production of
melatonin as a result.

Don't fool about with your head. Start your nighttime
routine by saying goodnight to your technology.
Avoid using electronics as much as you can in the
evening. Make sure to activate the red-light filter on
your phone before you even start your bedtime
routine so that it won't be as disruptive if you peek at
it accidentally.

7. Make time for meditation.
A regular meditation practice, like yoga, can enhance
the quality of your sleep. Instead of worrying about
not going to sleep, mindfulness meditation teaches

people to accept their thoughts and control their emotions, facilitating the beginning of sleep.

Simply closing your eyes and allowing yourself to concentrate on your thoughts and feelings is enough to engage in mindfulness meditation. Do not criticize your thoughts; simply observe them. Another type of meditation includes deep breathing or visualization. Numerous guided meditation activities are available for free on YouTube or mobile apps.

8. Read a quality book.
Reading before bed is a typical practice that starts in childhood. As part of the bedtime ritual, parents frequently read to their kids.

Avoid thrilling genres like mystery or action when adding reading to your sleep routine as an adult. The best books may have the least dramatic, even dull, plots.

9. Extend, breathe, and unwind.

By concentrating on your body and mindfully relaxing, relaxation techniques like deep breathing exercises and progressive muscle relaxation (PMR) can help you let go of physical and emotional strain. Simple stretches or a massage before bed can ease cramps, and a daily yoga regimen has been proven to enhance sleep quality.

You can greatly ease into sleep by doing some gentle yoga, stretching, and breathing techniques. Check out what works for you, then include it in your bedtime routine.

10. Set up your room.
Make changing your bedroom into a sleep haven a part of your bedtime routine. Make it a ritual to keep everything as quiet, dark, and cool as you can.

The temperature should be set between 60 and 71 degrees Fahrenheit. Disconnect any loud electronics. You should lower your blackout drapes and dim the lights. Clear the clutter and store items. Use an aromatherapy diffuser to enjoy your favorite perfume.

The last step of your evening regimen is to get into bed. Once your head touches the pillow, stop all activity and try to fall asleep. Make this the very last thing you do. Simply put, you want your brain to associate your bed with rest.

CHAPTER 6

TAKE VITAMINS

If you make an effort to eat a healthy diet, you may have some knowledge of the importance of consuming foods that are rich in essential vitamins and minerals. A balanced diet will give your body the vitamins and minerals it needs, which are necessary for optimal health. Healthy eating can be difficult for many people, so using a multivitamin and multimineral pill is a wonderful way to remain on track.

We have the information you need if you want to increase the number of vitamins in your diet. The best way to take vitamins and when to do so are discussed below.

What Sort of Vitamins Are Recommended?

Understanding the different types of vitamins is crucial before using vitamin supplements. Always with a health care expert before using supplements to ensure that they are good for you.

Vitamins are divided into two categories: fat-soluble vitamins and water-soluble vitamins (B-complex vitamins and C vitamins) (A, D, E, and K). Water-soluble vitamins dissolve in water and are not kept in the body; instead, they are often excreted in the urine. The distinction between these two groups is that fat-soluble vitamins dissolve in fat before being absorbed into the bloodstream.
Since the body doesn't store water-soluble vitamins, you could require them more frequently.

In addition, there is the issue of the form: is it gummy, chewable, swallowable, capsule, or tablet? A chewable or gummy vitamin can be a better choice for you if you have trouble swallowing pills or just don't enjoy doing it. Gummies and chewable frequently have sweet flavors and vibrant colors, which can add a little excitement to taking your regular supplements.

The type of vitamin you take can also be in question if you adhere to a certain diet. Before adding anything to your cart, please be sure to read the complete ingredient list as some supplements may include animal products.

When Should You Take Your Vitamins?

Knowing when to take your vitamins is equally as vital as understanding how to do so. Before having breakfast and beginning their day, many individuals choose to take their vitamins first thing in the morning. Some people could like a different hour of the day. The hardest challenge can occasionally be remembering to take vitamins every day, so think about developing a regular regimen that fits your lifestyle.

It is also important to handle fat-soluble versus water-soluble vitamins differently. Never take a supplement containing a fat-soluble vitamin on an empty stomach, such as vitamin E. There must be some fat present for our digestive systems to absorb vitamin E. In contrast to iron, which might conflict with some foods like cheese, yogurt, eggs, milk, spinach, tea, coffee, or whole-grain bread, vitamin E is a perfect supplement to take with meals.

Do you usually time your vitamin intake with your workouts? Some people contend that taking vitamins is best done after exercise rather than before because doing so may cause the vitamins to move around in your stomach and create gastric acid production, which results in heartburn and acid reflux.

CONCLUSION
It is crucial to keep in mind that a multivitamin cannot, under any circumstances, substitute for a nutritious, well-balanced diet. A multivitamin primarily serves the function of bridging nutritional gaps and offers only a small sample of the enormous variety of beneficial nutrients and substances naturally present in the diet. It is unable to provide

the fiber, flavor, and enjoyment of foods that are essential to a healthy diet. Multivitamins, however, can be crucial when dietary intake is insufficient to satisfy nutritional needs. In this situation, a pricey brand name is not required because even inexpensive store products will produce results.

CHAPTER 7

WORKING OUT REGULARLY

Any movement that engages your muscles and forces your body to burn calories is considered exercise. There are many different kinds of physical activity, to name a few: swimming, running, jogging, walking, and dancing. Numerous health advantages of exercise, both physically and emotionally, have been demonstrated.

Want to feel better, be more energetic, and even live longer? Just exercise.

Regular physical activity and exercise have many positive health effects that are difficult to deny. Everyone, regardless of age, sex, or physical ability, benefits from exercise.

BENEFITS OF EXERCISING

1. Exercise reduces weight
Exercise can assist sustain weight loss or prevent excessive weight gain. Calorie burn occurs during physical exertion. You burn more calories when you engage in more vigorous exercise.

Regular gym visits are important but don't stress if you can't find a significant amount of time to work out every day. Anything you do is preferable to doing nothing at all. Simply increase your daily activity to gain the benefits of exercise. Take the stairs instead of the elevator or work harder at your housework. The key is consistency.

2. Exercise fights illnesses and ailments
Is heart illness giving you pause? Want to lower your blood pressure? Whatever your present weight, exercising increases the "good" cholesterol known as high-density lipoprotein (HDL), and lowers the bad cholesterol known as triglycerides. Your blood continues to flow normally as a result of these two factors, lowering your risk of cardiovascular

problems. Numerous health issues and difficulties are prevented or managed by regular exercise, including:

Metabolic syndrome Stroke
Elevated blood pressure
Diabetes type 2
Depression\sAnxiety
Many different cancers
Arthritis\sFalls
Moreso, it can help with cognitive development and reduce the risk of dying from any cause.

3. Exercise lifts one's spirits
Need some emotional support? Or do you need to unwind after a demanding day? Exercise in the gym or a brisk walk can assist. Different brain chemicals are stimulated by physical activity, which may make you feel happier, more at ease, and less stressed. Regular exercise can also help you feel better about your appearance and yourself, which can increase your confidence and self-esteem.

4. Exercise Increases Vigor

Tired of doing housework or grocery shopping? Your muscle strength and endurance can both increase with regular exercise. Exercise helps your circulatory system function more effectively and distributes oxygen and nutrients to your tissues. Additionally, you have greater energy to complete daily tasks as your heart and lung health improves.

5. Exercise helps you sleep better
Struggling to fall asleep? You can sleep better, deeper, and fall asleep more quickly if you exercise regularly. Just remember to avoid exercising right before bedtime if you don't want to be too stimulated to sleep.

6. Exercise revitalizes your sexual life
Do you feel too worn out or unfit to appreciate intimate physical contact? Regular exercise can increase your energy levels and confidence in your physical attractiveness, which could enhance your sex life.

However, there is more to it than that. Regular exercise may increase arousal in women. Additionally, guys who frequently exercise are less likely than those who don't to experience erectile dysfunction issues.

7. Working out may be enjoyable and social! Physical activity and exercise can be joyful. They allow you the chance to relax, take in the outdoors, or just do things that make you happy. Additionally, engaging in physical activity might facilitate social interactions with loved ones or close friends.

So join a soccer team, go trekking, or take a dance lesson. Find a sport you like, and just start doing it. Bored? Try something new or engage in activities with loved ones or friends.

CHAPTER 8

PRACTICE DEEP BREATHING TECHNIQUES

You are breathing if you are reading this. Intriguingly, breathing is a subconscious or involuntary body function because we do it whether or not we're thinking about it, according to the book Human Biology written by Thompson Rivers University. However, if we are aware of our breathing patterns, we may also deliberately control our breathing. For instance, we can choose to regulate our breathing by making it faster or slower, or by taking shallower or deeper breaths.

What Purpose Does Breathing Serve?
Breathing happens in two stages: inhalation (taking in the air) and expiration (breathing out). The large, dome-shaped muscle called the diaphragm, which is situated between your lungs and your heart, contracts and descends when you inhale. The lungs expand into

the extra space that is created in the chest cavity as a result. The diaphragm relaxes as you exhale because there is less air in your lungs.

Because our bodies need oxygen to function—including for moving muscles, breaking down food, and even reading these words—breathing is crucial to life. Carbon dioxide is produced as a byproduct of these reactions and is eliminated by breathing. proper up arrow

BENEFITS OF DEEP BREATHING

Diaphragmatic breathing, abdominal breathing, belly breathing, and timed respiration are other synonyms for deep breathing. When you inhale deeply, your lungs are filled with air coming in from your nose, and your lower belly rises.

Deep breathing seems odd to many of us. This is due to several factors. One way that body image in our culture affects breathing is negative. Women (and males) frequently contract their stomach muscles because a flat tummy is regarded as beautiful. This hinders deep breathing and progressively normalizes shallow "chest breathing," which raises anxiety and stress levels.

Also, Deep breathing can help you manage or enhance, for example:

1. By reducing levels of stress and anxiety, gastrointestinal (GI) diseases including irritable bowel syndrome (IBS) can be treated.

2. Elevated blood pressure

3. By reducing stress and encouraging relaxation, mental health issues including depression, anxiety, and post-traumatic stress disorder (PTSD), as well as sleep disorders like insomnia, can be treated.

4. By reducing perceived stress, pelvic floor issues like overactive bladder can be prevented

5. Pulmonary illness with chronic obstruction (COPD) enhances breathing and quality of life for people with COPD It improves the quality of life, lung function, and hyperventilation in those with mild to moderate asthma

6. By lowering inflammation and psoriasis flare, it may be possible to treat skin disorders including eczema (atopic dermatitis).

7. By encouraging heart rate variability, which is regarded as a sign of heart health, autoimmune diseases like lupus and rheumatoid arthritis (RA) can be prevented.

8. Neurological diseases such as Parkinson's disease, which at its severe stages can lead to dysphagia and respiratory problems

9. Hot flashes, which have a high heart rate and other perimenopause symptoms that could be stressful

10. Type 2 diabetes is characterized by high blood sugar levels and oxidative stress, both of which advance the condition.

BREATHING EXERCISES

You can focus on your slow, deep breathing while using breath concentration, which also helps you to let go of distracting thoughts and feelings. If you frequently hold it in your stomach, it's extremely beneficial.

initial steps Locate a peaceful, cozy spot to sit or lie down. Take a regular breath first. Try taking a deep breath next: Take a slow, deep breath in through your nose, allowing your lower abdomen and chest to rise as you fill your lungs. Allow your belly to fully expand. Currently, slowly exhale through your mouth (or your nose, if that feels more natural).

Practice focusing on your breath. After completing the aforementioned stages, you can begin regularly practicing controlled breathing. Combine deep breathing with relaxing imagery and perhaps a focal

word or phrase while you sit comfortably with your
eyes closed.

CHAPTER 9

EMPLOY POSITIVE THINKING/ATTITUDE

While it's simple to sink into a rut as a result of one bad event, it's also simple to turn your attention elsewhere and concentrate on the pleasant experiences.

Being optimistic about circumstances, relationships, and oneself is what is meant by having a good attitude. Even in the most challenging circumstances, those with positive attitudes maintain optimism and perceive the best. People with negative attitudes, on the other hand, could be more pessimistic and disagreeable, and they frequently anticipate the worst in challenging circumstances. Having a positive outlook can provide you with the tools you need to deal with stress more healthily, even while it won't necessarily make you feel less anxious.

Having a positive attitude involves more than just always having a smile on your face. It involves keeping a positive outlook and attitude even while everything around you is in complete disarray. Positive and negative thoughts are considered to have a similar effect on your mind as a healthy or unhealthy diet has on your physical health. Positive ideas will help you witness great improvements in the world around you.

When you begin to think positively, your mind gets free of all negative ideas, and you begin to perceive the world in a new way. You will no longer blame yourself or other people. You will have complete emotional control and make an effort to learn something from every setback you encounter.

REASONS TO ADOPT POSITIVE THINKING

1. Happiness: It is well known that happiness and a positive outlook go hand in hand. Happiness is a mental state that comes from the inside and is not

reliant on outside circumstances. Positive thinking will bring harmony and happiness into your life. Simply put, no matter what circumstances you are in, you may be happy right now if you have a positive mindset.

2. Self-assurance: You'll start to feel better about yourself after you adopt an optimistic outlook. Your confidence and inner strength will increase as a result of treating yourself with more love and respect. You'll overcome your self-limiting beliefs and take on fresh tasks.

3. A stronger immune system: Those who have a positive outlook are vivacious, active, and healthy. Positive thinking has a beneficial impact on your health as well, reducing stress and enhancing your general welfare. Even when you are sick, your body heals more quickly.

4. More focused: By adopting a positive outlook, you can establish emotional equilibrium, which aids the brain's healthy operation. You develop the ability to

maintain attention, which enables you to make wise choices in difficult circumstances.

10 WAYS TO ADOPT POSITIVE THINKING

1. Begin a journal of appreciation:
Why not remind yourself of this every day? There are so many things in life for which to be grateful. A thankfulness diary is a great tool for maintaining a cheerful outlook each day. You list at least three things in your day for which you are grateful once a day. They can be tiny, like spotting an adorable dog on the way to work, or big, like obtaining a job offer for your dream position. They can also be things that happened to you on that particular day, like getting yourself a huge latte, or things that are a constant in your life, like having a loving family.

You are free to write whatever you wish. It's only important that you keep in mind to express gratitude each day. You can cultivate a more optimistic view by retraining your mind to consider all the positive aspects of your life.

2. Reward yourself with daily self-care:
Taking care of your physical and emotional wellness is always crucial. When you have a full-time job that demands you to contact people all the time in high-stress circumstances, whether they be customers, prospects, coworkers, or supervisors, it can feel overwhelming. Take a step back and reward yourself with something unique to keep moving forward with a good outlook. Even if it sounds great, self-care doesn't usually entail a romantic nighttime bath with candles and a bottle of wine.

Think about how you can relax, decompress, and spend some "you" time. A face mask, a movie, baking, reading, contacting a friend, ordering takeout, or even just saying "no" to plans and staying in are a few possibilities. You should develop the practice of exercising something every day, no matter what it is. You can assure a more positive attitude when you're working long hours by allowing yourself these breaks.

3. Get a good start each morning:
If you put a positive attitude into practice as soon as you get up in the morning, it will be simpler to keep it all day. The dreaded alarm sound can frequently cause annoyance, which leads to a bad attitude for the rest of the day.

Instead, consider some strategies to improve your morning, especially if you're not a morning person. Think about rising an hour or earlier than normal. This necessitates an earlier bedtime as well! Give yourself time to indulge in the activities you enjoy but may not always find the time for, such as going for a run, taking a hot shower, sipping coffee, and truly preparing breakfast (granola bars and frozen waffles do not qualify). Start your morning doing something you love while savoring a home-cooked meal. Put on your preferred music or TV. You could even grab a book. You'll undoubtedly arrive at work in a better mood when your morning is more productive and less hurried. Your day will be infused with that early radiance, and the cycle might repeat itself.

4. Refrain from gossiping:
Many people make their living by spreading rumors.
But even if something is true, saying it behind
someone's back when you wouldn't say it in front of
them is wrong. Gossip creates an unsteady, risky, and
unpleasant atmosphere at work. Because if you're
distributing false information about your coworkers,
they're likely doing the same about you.

Even though avoiding gossip can be challenging,
resist the urge to participate. If someone tries to
share a shocking anecdote about a coworker, politely
decline and say you'd prefer not to take part.
Although it may seem strange, you'll notice that you
feel lighter when you're not dragging around secrets.
Additionally, you might feel more assured that others
are keeping their mouths shut about you when you
aren't talking about them. And that's a cause for
optimism.

5. Laugh out loud more:

The most effective treatment is humor. Laughter has fantastic immediate effects on your body and mindset. The Mayo Clinic states that laughter can boost endorphin levels, reduce stress, and let the tension out.

Laughter and the pleasant ideas that go along with it have the potential to release neuropeptides in the long run that combat stress and other major ailments. It can also make you happier and assist you in overcoming challenges. By telling more jokes, you can find comedy in potentially unpleasant workplace situations while also preparing your body and mind for a more upbeat approach.

6. Enjoy genuine breaks:
It can occasionally be challenging to find time for a significant break during a hectic, eight-hour workday. That entails leaving the office, eating, and putting away all paperwork associated with the job. You should never feel as though your right to a break is in danger because it is permitted by law.

Eight hours of nonstop work can leave you feeling drained and agitated. Even a short break of 30 minutes will help you feel more energized and inspired to finish the day's job. Give yourself some time to replenish your optimism, and you'll end the day feeling better.

7. Plan an exciting after-work activity:
Even though you might be exhausted after a long day at work, having plans for after 5 p.m. can make the day seem a bit more promising. A fun-filled evening with your loved ones, workplace, or friends can help the day fly by.

You don't necessarily have to go out for dinner or drinks as part of your plans. Even making plans for a Netflix marathon might make your work more enjoyable. Making your days more than just "work" is the goal. You can discover a good method to balance your personal and professional lives by scheduling some leisure time several days a week.

8. Make time to meditate:

Meditation can significantly reduce stress and anxiety as well as enhance one's mental and spiritual well-being. For those who work in high-pressure environments, such as in customer support or service, proper meditation can reduce anxiety at work.

A daily meditation practice can be started in just five minutes. Clarify your thoughts and practice deep breathing. You may establish balance in your life and let go of any tension or negativity you may be experiencing with the help of easy techniques like these.

9. Pay attention to the long term rather than the immediate:
Your first instinct may be to defend yourself when a dispute arises, whether it is with a coworker or a client. It's wise to desire to keep yourself safe and get respect. But the more disputes you become involved in, the more negativity will surround your life.

Instead, take a moment to stand back and consider the scenario from the viewpoint of a neutral person. Will my involvement in this fight end up helping me in the long run? Or will it just add to the tension and negativity we already feel?

A consumer will frequently just be having a poor day or a stressed-out coworker. You can learn empathy instead of reacting angrily. By doing so, you might be able to solve the issue at its core and make a good impression by wrapping up the discussion.

10. Play tunes that reflect your mood:
Ironically, listening to depressing music could improve your mood. A survey found that many people listen to depressing music to lift their spirits. Sad music is often referred to as "beautiful," which improves mood. Sad songs can also evoke strong memories, serve as a diversion from terrible circumstances, and convey important ideas.

According to a different study, listening to sad music may make people feel better since doing so makes melancholy seem more happy and rewarding. Therefore, listening to depressing music during or after a long, arduous labor may simply improve your attitude. Play some Adele and watch your bad mood vanish.

When you put the aforementioned advice into practice, your attitude will noticeably change. You'll also discover that it manifests itself in your behavior. Look at some illustrations of what having a positive attitude might look like in your daily life and at work.

CONCLUSION
Positive affirmations are a powerful tool for teaching your mind to think positively. Repeating them will help your mind build a positive attitude. You may combat negative ideas and cultivate optimism in yourself by reading motivational and inspiring quotes every day.
Any negative incident should be approached with optimism, and you should try to draw a good conclusion from it.

Keep in mind that your thoughts influence your moods and behavior. You should therefore instantly replace any negative thoughts that enter your head with positive ones. Even if things are bad, having an optimistic outlook will help you get through the challenging period without too much difficulty.
No matter the circumstances, commit to being upbeat. Instead of worrying if things aren't going your way, keep working toward your objectives with an optimistic outlook, and you'll soon start to see wonderful results!

CHAPTER 10

HEALTHY EATING

Depending on who you ask, "healthy eating" can mean different things to different people. Everyone appears to have an opinion on the healthiest diet, including medical professionals, wellness influencers, coworkers, and family members. Additionally, online nutrition articles can be extremely perplexing due to their inconsistent and frequently erroneous advice and guidelines.

If all you want to do is eat in a way that is good for you, this makes it difficult. The truth is that eating a balanced diet doesn't have to be difficult. It is possible to eat the foods you love and still fuel your body. After all, food should not be feared, tallied, weighed, or tracked; rather, it should be enjoyed.

Healthy eating is not about imposing severe restrictions, maintaining an unattainable level of thinness, or depriving yourself of your favorite foods. Instead, it's about increasing your health, mood, and energy levels while feeling fantastic.

Eating healthy doesn't have to be difficult. You're not alone if you feel overloaded by the contradicting nutrition and diet recommendations available. It appears that for every expert who says a particular cuisine is healthy, there are two more who suggest the exact opposite. In actuality, although some particular foods or minerals have been found to have a positive impact on mood, your entire dietary pattern is what matters most. Real food should always be preferred above processed food as the cornerstone of a balanced diet. Eating food that is as close to how nature intended it can have a profound impact on how you feel, look, and think.

One of the most significant things you can do to safeguard your health is to eat a healthy, balanced diet. Lifestyle choices and behaviors like eating a nutritious diet and exercising regularly can prevent up to 80% of early heart disease and stroke. Your risk

of heart disease and stroke can be decreased by
eating a balanced diet:
decreasing your cholesterol
decreasing blood pressure
controlling your blood sugar while assisting you in
managing your body weight.

A BALANCED DIET CONSISTS OF:

1. Consuming a lot of fruit and veggies
One of the most significant dietary practices is this.
Fruit and vegetables are rich in nutrients
(antioxidants, vitamins, minerals, and fiber) and help
you maintain a healthy weight by making you feel
satisfied for longer periods.
At every meal and snack, place fruit and vegetables
on half of your plate.

2. Opting for whole-grain meal options
Brown or wild rice, quinoa, oatmeal, whole-wheat
bread, crackers, and hulled barley are examples of
whole-grain foods. The entire grain is used in their

preparation. Because they are high in protein, fiber, and B vitamins, whole-grain foods will keep you feeling fuller for longer.

Instead of refined or processed grains like white bread and pasta, choose whole-grain options. A quarter of your plate should be made up of whole-grain items.

3. Eating Protein-rich Foods

Legumes, nuts, seeds, tofu, fortified soy beverages, fish, shellfish, eggs, poultry, lean red meats, including wild game, low-fat milk, low-fat yogurts, low-fat kefir, and low-fat and low-sodium cheeses are examples of foods high in protein.

Building and maintaining bones, muscles, and skin both require protein. daily protein consumption

Eat more plant-based foods and try to eat at least two servings of fish every week. Protein is abundant in dairy products. Opt for bland, lower-fat selections. Protein-rich foods should take up a quarter of your plate.

4. Reducing your intake of highly and ultra-processed meals
Foods that have undergone extensive processing also referred to as ultra-processed foods differ significantly from their original food sources. Important nutrients including vitamins, minerals, and fiber are frequently lost during processing while salt and sugar are added. Fast food, hot dogs, chips, cookies, frozen pizzas, deli meats, white rice, and white bread are a few examples of processed foods. Some meals with little processing are OK. These are foods that have been marginally modified but include only a little amount of industrially produced additives. Almost all of the nutrients in minimally processed foods are still present. Bagged salad, frozen fruit and vegetables, eggs, milk, cheese, flour, brown rice, oil, and dry herbs are a few examples. When we suggest that you avoid processed foods, we are not referring to these minimally processed foods.

5. Making Water Your Preferred Beverage
Without adding calories to the diet, water improves hydration and supports health.

Energy drinks, fruit drinks, 100% fruit juice, soft drinks, and flavored coffees are among the sugary beverages that have a lot of sugar but little to no nutritional benefit. Without realizing it, it is simple to consume empty calories, which causes weight gain. Avoid fruit juice, even if it is made entirely of fruit. Fruit juice offers some of the same vitamins and minerals as fruit, but it also has more sugar and less fiber. Fruit juice shouldn't be substituted for fruits in your diet. Fruits should be consumed, not drunk, by Canadians.

If there isn't any safe drinking water available, try coffee, tea, unsweetened low-fat milk, and previously boiled water to relieve your thirst.

It could take some time to establish a positive relationship with eating. You're not alone if you don't have a positive relationship with eating. Eating disorders or tendencies toward disordered eating are common. It's crucial to receive the appropriate care if you have concerns that you may have one of these disorders.You need the proper equipment if you want to establish a positive relationship with food. Here are some practical suggestions to help you start eating healthily:

1. Give plant-based food priority:
Your diet should be primarily composed of plant foods including fruits, vegetables, legumes, and nuts. Consider including these foods, particularly fruits and vegetables, at each meal and snack.

2. Cook meals at home:
Having a varied diet is made easier by cooking at home. If you're used to eating out or ordering takeout, start with cooking only one or two meals per week.
routine grocery shopping You're more likely to prepare healthy meals and snacks if your kitchen is stocked with nutritious ingredients. Make one or two weekly grocery runs to ensure you have a supply of wholesome foods. Recognize that your diet won't be flawless. Progress, not perfection, is what matters. Wherever you are, accept yourself. Cooking one handmade, nutrient-dense meal per week if you now eat out every night is a major improvement.

3. "Cheat Days" Are Not Permitted:
Having "cheat days" or "cheat meals" regularly
indicates that your diet is out of balance. There is no
need to cheat once you realize that all foods may be a
part of a balanced diet.

4. Avoid drinks that are sugar-sweetened:
As much as you can, avoid drinking sugary beverages
like soda, energy drinks, and sweetened coffee.
Drinking sugary beverages frequently can be bad for
your health.

5. Select satiating foods:
When you're hungry, you should aim to eat satisfying,
healthy foods rather than trying to consume as few
calories as possible. Choose meals and snacks that are
high in protein and fiber to keep you full.

6. Consume real food:
Whole foods including vegetables, fruits, legumes,
nuts, seeds, whole grains, and protein sources like

eggs and fish should make up the majority of a balanced diet.

7. Hydrate properly:
Healthy nutrition includes staying hydrated, and the easiest way to do so is with water. Get a reusable water bottle and flavor it with fruit slices or a touch of lemon if you're not used to drinking water.

8. Respect your distastes:
Don't eat something if you've tried it multiple times and don't like it. There are lots of nutritious foods available as alternatives. Just because something is seen as healthy doesn't mean you have to consume it.

CONCLUSION
Making a few minor adjustments can help you start eating healthier if you're interested. Balanced diets are often high in nutrient-dense foods, low in highly processed foods, and made up of full meals and snacks, however, healthy eating may look a little different for everyone.

CHAPTER 11

MAINTAIN HEALTHY WEIGHT

Maintaining a healthy weight is essential for overall health and well-being. It's important to remember that a healthy weight isn't just about looking good; it's about feeling good too.

When it comes to maintaining a healthy weight, it's not just about dieting or exercising – it's about making lifestyle changes that can help you achieve and maintain your desired weight.

Here are some tips to help you maintain a healthy weight:

1. Eat a balanced diet: A balanced diet is the cornerstone of a healthy lifestyle and helps you maintain a healthy weight. Make sure you're getting a variety of foods from all the food groups, including

fruits, vegetables, whole grains, lean proteins, and healthy fats.

2. Get regular physical activity: Regular physical activity can help you maintain a healthy weight and prevent weight gain. Aim for at least 150 minutes of moderate-intensity physical activity per week.

3. Monitor your portions: It's important to be aware of how much you're eating. Use smaller plates, avoid second helpings, and be mindful of how much food you're consuming.

4. Control your cravings: Many of us have cravings for unhealthy foods. To maintain a healthy weight, you'll need to control those cravings and make better choices.

5. Get enough sleep: Sleep is essential for good health, and it can also help you maintain a healthy weight. Aim for 7-8 hours of sleep per night.

6. Avoid stress: Stress can lead to unhealthy habits, including overeating. Make sure you're taking time to relax and manage your stress levels.

7. Stay hydrated: Drinking enough water is essential for good health and helps you maintain a healthy weight. Aim for 8-10 glasses of water a day.